Definitive Trichology's
Complete Guide to Beautiful, Healthy Hair

Angela Adams McGhee

Published by
Definitive Formulations, LLC
3900 Dave Ward Drive STE1900 #276
Conway, AR 72034

Edited by
Katti Bowen

Library of Congress Control Number: 2015906466

ISBN-13: 978-0-692-42572-5

DEDICATION

Now unto Him who is able to keep you from falling, and
to present you faultless before the presence of his glory
with exceeding joy, to the only wise God our Savior,
be glory and majesty, dominion and power,
both now and forever, Amen.
Jude 1:24-25, *King James Version*

To Herman and Emma Adams
Parents who never failed to believe and support,

To Marla Nicole
Be the high tower among consecrated people,

To Monica Elise
Be the advisor consecrated to God,

To all my family and friends for the encouragement to
pursue my dreams.

CONTENTS

ACKNOWLEDGMENTS

The International Association of Trichologists (IAT) under the leadership of David Salinger, helped greatly enrich my knowledge of the subject of hair care.

i

INTRODUCTION

If I had to guess, I'm thinking this isn't the first book on hair care that you have read. My plan is for this to be the last one you need. In reading this book, you will get all the information you need about hair structure, types, and care. What sets this book apart is that we'll also cover nutrition, medical conditions, and other factors that can't be ignored if you want healthy hair. At the end of each chapter you will be asked to make notes in chapter 7. The information you record will help you create a customized hair health plan.

There is a chance that you don't know me or why you should read my book, so here's my background. By formal education, I am a chemist who specializes in cosmetic chemistry and the formulation of hair, skin, and fragrance products for my company Definitive Formulations, LLC. We've worked with clients across the country on products for their salons, spas, and boutiques.

Additionally, I am a certified Trichologist through the International Association of Trichologists. I practice under the company name Definitive Trichology. You'll learn about Trichology, the study of the hair and scalp, and how various factors affect your hair and scalp. We'll also discuss when to end the home remedies and to seek professional help. Join me on the journey to beautiful, healthy hair.

Angela

CHAPTER 1
THE BASICS:
HAIR & SKIN STRUCTURE

It may be tempting, but don't skip ahead. If you truly want to improve your hair, you will need to know its structure and function. This will be painless – I promise.

SKIN STRUCTURE & FUNCTION

Why start here? Hair is an appendage (or attachment) to the skin. The skin is the home and foundation for every hair and is vital to its healthy existence. In fact, skin is the largest organ of the human body. It helps regulate body temperature, provides protection for the entire body, and contains unique cells that provide sensory information about the environment and substances that may potentially harm the body.

The skin consists of 3 main layers: the epidermis (the part you see and feel), the dermis, and below the dermis is the subcutaneous (or fat) layer. In most areas of the body, skin is merely 4 millimeters thick.

A key point to note is that the dermis layer of the skin contains the hair follicles which are surrounded by a complex system of blood vessels and nerves. This foundation is how the body supplies nutrients to the hair bulb in order to produce the cells that eventually form the hair strand. The skin also contains the sebaceous glands that help supply sebum, also known as oil, to the hair and scalp as well as the sweat glands which help regulate body temperature.

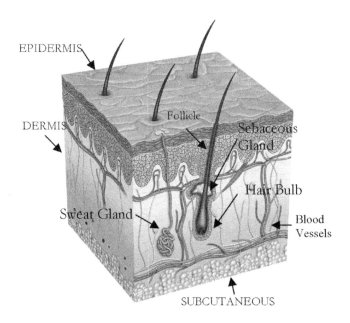

HAIR STRUCTURE AND FUNCTION

The hair of a human has many functions depending on the location of the hair. On the scalp, hair helps protect the head from impact, provides cover from the elements, can help keep the head warm, and not to mention, it's our "crowning glory." Eyebrows help keep sweat and debris from the eyes. Eyelashes detect potential hazards to the eye and help keep debris from entering the eye. Of course, our focus will be on the hair of the scalp.

So, let's talk structure. I am sure you are familiar with the terms cuticle, cortex, and medulla, but let's discuss each one in more detail.

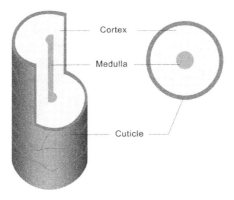

The cuticle of the hair is the outer surface. It is made of overlapping elongated cells. For treatments to effect the structure of the hair, they will have to penetrate the cuticle. When the cuticle is smooth and intact, hair looks healthy. For straight hair, a smooth cuticle helps achieve a beautiful shine; however, when the cuticle is damaged hair feels rough as you slide fingers from root to end of the hair strand. In very curly or wavy hair there is a natural "lift" of the cuticle where hair makes a sharp change in direction to form a ringlet or curl. This feature can make these hair types more vulnerable to damage, but it can also lead to the use of the term "coarse" as a hair type. The cuticle takes the abuse of styling. In fact, the concept of "teasing" the hair required the reverse combing of hair from end to root, which goes against the natural direction of the cuticle. This causes the lifting of the cuticle and the effect of tangling the hair.

Beneath the cuticle is the cortex. It is made of lengthwise fibers that give hair its ability to stretch (elasticity) and it is the basis of the curl pattern of the hair. Within the cortex, lengthwise fibers are held together by 3 types of chemical bonds that give hair its strength: hydrogen bonds, ionic bonds and disulfide bonds. Each bond type contributes to approximately one-third of the strength of the hair. When hair is wet, both hydrogen and ionic bonds are broken and then reform when hair is dry. Since wet hair has two-thirds of its strength compromised, it is important to be gentle with wet hair. The cortex is also where the pigment is deposited that creates the hair color. Gray hair is the result of no pigment being deposited into the growing strand.

In the very center of the hair strand is the medulla. In hair types with very small diameter strands, the medulla may not be present at all.

At the base of the strand of hair is the bulb which is surrounded by a dense network of capillaries and nerves. While the hair is in its growth phase, the body supplies nutrients to the hair through the bulb. Scalp hair grows approximately 0.35 millimeters per day and continues to grow anywhere from 2 to 6 years[1]. The length of time each strand remains in the growth (anagen) phase determines how much length can potentially accumulate. When the anagen phase ends, the nerve structure goes dormant and the capillaries collapse. This is why it doesn't cause pain when a hair falls out like it does when you pluck an intact one. After the growth cycle is complete, the hair is in a resting state, called catagen, for approximately 1 week. Then the hair is shed during the telogen phase which lasts up to 3 months.

While the hair is awaiting removal by combing, brushing, etc. the new hair begins growth in the bottom of the follicle and will ultimately push the "old" unshed hair out as it accumulates length. At any point in time, approximately 85% of hair is in the anagen phase, 1% is in the catagen phase, and 14% is in the telogen phase[2]. This equates to approximately 70 to 100 hairs per day lost, depending on the total number of follicles you have. Fortunately, every hair is on an individual cycle, otherwise we would go bald every after every telogen cycle!

Each follicle is also capable of producing different types of hair. Infants are usually born with fine hair called lanugo. After several months, or at birth in some ethnicities, vellus hairs appear. Vellus hairs are still fine hairs but are often pigmented depending on genetics. The follicle may later be capable of producing terminal hair that appears on the scalp, eyebrows, and eyelashes. The post-puberty hair on the face, underarms, chest, back, arms, legs and pubic hair are all terminal hairs. Terminal hair is larger in diameter than the previous types discussed and pigmented according to the genetics of the person.

In case you're wondering how a growing hair stays in the follicle if it's only attached at the root – there's more to it than that. The follicle surface in contact with the hair strand near the bulb is called the inner root sheath. The inner root sheath has its own cuticle which interlocks with the cuticle of the growing hair strand, thus keeping the hair secured in the follicle.

Angela Adams McGhee

CHAPTER 2:
BETTER SKIN & HAIR
FROM THE INSIDE OUT

In summary from chapter 1, skin is an organ and hair and nails are appendages, or attachments. While your hair is important, it's not necessary for the body to fully function.

Why stress this point? Your body's command center, also known as the brain, places a priority on what is necessary to maintain your life and in order to do that organs come first. This means hair, skin, and nails are not maintained as a group by a daily supplement.

In this chapter, we're going to learn how to maintain the necessities of the body so that it can then adequately support healthy hair and nails.

Priority 1 is to maintain the skin. Unlike hair, which has a resting phase, skin continually regenerates itself. Considering that skin covers your entire body, we're talking about millions of cells. It is estimated that about 20%[3] of your body's protein intake is used to fuel this process.

Aside from startling scenes in horror movies, you probably don't know of anyone having skin fall off due to a nutritional deficiency. However, you may know many people who notice brittle hair and nails and even hair loss after crash dieting or poor diet (even if they don't know that's the cause).

Let's begin with nutrition. We all know that it is recommended that we eat breakfast, lunch, dinner and healthy snacks. We also know that we should eat from the four major food groups: milk/dairy, fruit/vegetable, grains and meat. However, today we are immersed in a culture that touts gluten-free, lactose-intolerant, low-carb, low-fat, vegetarianism, and veganism. With all these dietary restrictions, it's easy to get confused so we're going to start with proteins, vitamins, and minerals.

PROTEIN

It is the building block of every cell in the body. A lack of protein isn't just a hair problem, it's a health problem. Historically, the food group system has suggested the "meat" group as the ideal source for protein. This logic is based on the knowledge that most animals eat grains of various types, then their systems are able to make other amino acids, the components of protein. The animal meat supplies what is called a "complete" protein. The term "complete protein" means they have a wide variety of the amino acids your body needs. Vegans and vegetarians can live a very healthy lifestyle without meat provided their diet includes a wide enough variety of beans and vegetables to give them the proteins they need.

In the US, the Recommended Daily Allowance (RDA) is as follows[4]:

Children (ages 1-3)	13 grams/day
Children (ages 4-8)	19 grams/day
Children (ages 9-13)	34 grams/day
Girls/Women (ages 14-70+)	46 grams/day
Boys (ages 14-18)	52 grams/day
Men (ages 19-70+)	56 grams/day

You can take in protein from this list of sources:
Milk, Greek yogurt, chicken, beef, fish, eggs, beans (i.e. pinto beans, black-eyed peas, etc.), tofu, soybeans,

chicken, fish, beef and some cuts of pork. Bacon is a relatively poor choice given its fat to protein ratio.

Honestly, if you aren't a fan of the protein sources listed above, you can find some bars (the ones with 20g+ of protein) or even purchase the flavored whey powders to add to a fruit smoothie. Just remember, you will likely meet your daily protein intake needs by eating a good protein source at each meal.

Organic eggs, meat, and vegetable choices are becoming readily available at all price points. Choosing organic options minimizes the use of chemical fertilizers, growth-enhancing hormones, and other impurities that can introduce toxins into the body that may cause a variety of adverse health effects.

VITAMINS

In addition to your protein intake, vitamins play a vital role in your health and the health of your hair. Vitamins are classified as either fat soluble (excess amounts are stored in the tissues in the body) or water soluble (the body uses what it needs and the rest drains out with your "fluid elimination.")

We'll begin with fat-soluble vitamins. It is important to make sure you don't over consume these if you choose to take supplements to boost your vitamin intake. Since they can be stored in the tissues of the body it is possible to "overdose" by consuming excess amounts from supplements.

- Vitamin K – assists in blood clotting and therefore bruise healing. Found in leafy, deep green veggies (iceberg lettuce does not apply)
- Vitamin A – helps improve and maintain eyesight, bone development and skin health. In fact, topical Vitamin A is used to treat acne and refine skin texture. Vitamin A works with zinc to help promote healthy hair. Carrots, sweet potatoes, spinach, broccoli and pumpkin are rich sources of

vitamin A.

- Vitamin D is one of the most diagnosed deficiencies today in people of all shades of skin color. Vitamin D can easily be manufactured in the skin with exposure to sunlight; however, today we know that sun exposure leads to tanning (which is skin damage) and can cause premature aging of the skin and even cancer. It is recommended that we wear sunscreen regularly and avoid excessive exposure to the sun. Vitamin D is also vital to bone formation and health. What you may not know is that it is linked to hair health and even your mood regulation. Vitamin D is found in fortified milk, eggs, fish and liver. If you are choosing organic milk, read the nutrition label to verify if the milk has been fortified with Vitamin D. If you need to supplement, Vitamin D3 is more easily metabolized. Follow your doctor's recommended dosage.

- Vitamin E – is a powerful antioxidant. This means that it fights free radicals (cells that have lost an electron and cause damage to other cells in the body). Vitamin E is key in healthy cell development, including hair cells. Vitamin E can be found in cold processed oils, soybeans, and raw nuts.

Moving on, water soluble vitamins include the B-family and Vitamin C. The Vitamin B family includes: B1 (thiamine), B2 (riboflavin), B3 (niacin), B5 (pantothenic acid), B6 (pyroxidine), B12 (cobalamine), biotin, and folate.

You probably noticed biotin on the list. Often touted as the holy grail of hair, skin, and nail growth; sadly, there just isn't enough scientific evidence to prove it fuels massive hair growth. Also consider that it is in the "water soluble" vitamin group which means your massive dose in supplement form is literally being flushed down the toilet.

- The B-family serves a host of functions in the body. They can best be summarized as being key to cell formation, functionality, and metabolism. The B vitamins can be found in Brewer's yeast (a supplement with all the B vitamins), eggs, liver, meat, fish, and whole grains.

- Vitamin C – it's an antioxidant (like vitamin E) that works on important structures, like collagen formation in the skin. It is also necessary for the formation of the sulfur bonds that give hair its strength. Found in citrus fruit, strawberries, broccoli, and many more fruits and vegetables.

So, why the lesson on vitamins? Simply put, they are vital to the healthy functioning of your body. When your system is functioning at its best, energy and nutrients are made available for hair and nail growth.

MINERALS

The human body uses minerals either to perform a direct function or to be present for certain reactions to occur. When it comes to the complex process of hair growth, many minerals are necessary but we will cover a few of the vital ones.

- Iron – helps with red blood cell transport of hemoglobin. Deficiencies in iron can result in anemia which can cause hair loss. Iron and Vitamin C work together in hair health. Iron can be found in liver, meat, eggs, and whole grains.

- Manganese – helps grow connective tissue (like collagen and the inner root sheath). Deficiencies can cause slow hair and nail growth. It can be found in seeds, beans, eggs, and whole grains.

- Silicon – contributes to the strength of connective tissue and helps with bone strength. It can be found in rice, soybeans, and seafood.

- Zinc – plays a major part in the enzymes that help in digestion. Poor digestion leads to poor absorption of vitamins, minerals and protein. Therefore, the body is still nutritionally deficient and hair loss can occur. Zinc is found in spinach, Brewer's yeast, various protein sources and whole grains[5].

When it comes to minerals, it is better not to self-supplement. Meaning, more is not better and may even be harmful to your health. Many minerals have a direct relationship with other minerals. For example, zinc and copper must be in the correct ratio for proper creation of thyroid hormone. Over consuming zinc or copper could, therefore, lead to thyroid issues.

In order to have healthy hair, you will need to drink plenty of water. What's the connection between water and hair growth? Water is used to make blood which is obviously vital to the human body. Your body also needs water to aid the digestive process. Inadequate water can lead to constipation and other digestion and excretion issues. Digestion issues can lead to malabsorption of the proteins, vitamins, and minerals needed to keep your body (and hair production) at its optimal performance; therefore, water is needed for healthy hair. For those of us who don't regularly like to drink pure water, start slowly by reducing one soda or other beverage per day and replacing it with water. Keep increasing water until you get at least 64 ounces per day. (No, it doesn't count when the Coca-Cola® bottling company uses it to make your favorite soda!)

In summary, save on the supplements, unless you want to take Brewer's yeast in a capsule. (Trust me, you might not enjoy the aftertaste of the powder - yuck) A healthy diet will fuel the healthy hair growth you desire.

As for speeding up hair growth, the only sound advice here is something that will come as no surprise. The only way to speed up hair growth is to perhaps speed your metabolism. The only SAFE way to increase metabolism is through a nutritious diet and effective exercise program. NOTE: please see a doctor before beginning any exercise or starting a supplement plan. Your physician can ensure there won't be any negative side effects with medications you may be taking or issues with any existing health conditions you may have.

CHAPTER 3
HAIR TYPES &
HOW TO DETERMINE YOURS

In order to truly improve the health of your hair, you must know much more than whether you're normal, oily or dry. There are several characteristics you must understand in order to achieve better hair. We will cover each of the following in detail: porosity, density, diameter, elasticity, and curl pattern. While you can't necessarily change all of them, they play an essential role in everything from product selection to chemical treatment type, and time needed to properly chemically process the hair.

POROSITY
Porosity is simply how easy it is for moisture (and chemicals) to penetrate the hair shaft. This characteristic is genetically linked but the condition of your hair also plays a huge role in determining porosity. For example, those who seem to have chronically dry hair despite moisturizing and have frizzy hair at the slightest increase in humidity are likely to have highly porous hair. This means that the cuticle freely allows humidity in and freely lets moisture out, causing a need for daily moisturizing.

In contrast, hair with low porosity can be difficult to moisturize. While it doesn't readily react to humidity, it can be "resistant" to chemical processing – requiring higher strength of chemicals or longer processing time.

So, how do you determine the porosity of your hair? Here's a simple test to perform next time you shampoo your hair. After rinsing the shampoo thoroughly from your hair, save a few stands before conditioning and let them dry overnight on a paper towel. Next, complete the following steps:

Step 1: Fill a clear glass with plain tap water.

Step 2: Gently lay a single strand across the top of the surface of the water.

Step 3: Record the time it takes for the hair to sink below the surface.

The following results will indicate the porosity of your hair:

- < 1 minute   (highly porous hair)
- Up to 1.5 minutes   (normal porosity)
- >1.5 minutes   (low porosity)

Once you have determined your hair's porosity, turn to chapter 7 and capture it on your Customized Hair Health Plan.

Dealing with highly porous hair can be frustrating, but this treatment can give your hair some stability.

"Moisture sealing" the hair is a two step process that allows you to add moisture with a water based product and seal it with an emollient (oil based product). This process can be done on either wet or dry hair.

Step 1: Apply a rich, moisturizing crème throughout the hair.

Step 2: Apply an oil based pomade over the hair in sections.

This method works if you are air drying hair or thermally styling hair. If you don't plan to blow dry or thermally straighten your hair, add the moisturizer and follow with the pomade. If you are thermally styling, perform step 1 before hair dries, then apply pomade from step 2 sparingly before blow drying. (Less is needed because the heat from the styling tool will melt and distribute the oils.)

Why does this process work? The water based product adds moisture and a pomade type product forms a barrier that helps keep the water from easily evaporating into dry air or water in the air from entering the hair shaft as easily as it does when this method isn't used. See chapter 6 for guidance on how to select the products that help you get the best results.

For those with low porosity, hair generally takes longer to wet. If you experience dryness, you will need to make sure your moisturizer has a pH value between 4.5-5.5 to help it penetrate your hair shaft. You can also do moisture sealing, but you will likely need a lighter weight pomade than your highly porous friends.

While you can't change your low porosity hair, make sure you understand and share this with your stylist who must take this into account when planning your perm, relaxer, bleach, or color service. If they don't understand why you are telling them about the porosity of your hair - leave immediately.

If you ignore this warning, you have greatly increased your odds of having over/underprocessed hair.

As mentioned previously, damage to the hair's cuticle can cause the hair to become more porous. This is why proper processing, maintenance, and styling techniques are so important. Turn to chapter 7 to record your porosity rating for future use in the Customized Hair Health Plan.

DIAMETER

Diameter is the relative thickness of a strand of hair. Diameter is important because it helps define the density of hair. Typically, you cannot alter diameter as it is genetically determined. Products that say they make your hair thicker are taking one of two approaches. One approach is to use a very low pH or high pH to swell the hair shaft. The other approach is to use polymers or fixatives to put "space" between the hair fibers. As we will discuss in chapter 5, changes in your system can cause hair loss and the new hair may initially grow back with a smaller diameter. During the next growth cycle, if the body condition is back to normal, the hair will likely return to its original diameter.

One additional thing about diameter is that it is a factor in the strength of hair. It has been said that a healthy strand of hair is stronger than a piece of copper wire of the same diameter. Asian hair generally has of the largest diameter hair. This characteristic contributes to the strength and vitality of hair that is a favorite in the manufacture of human hair extensions and wigs.

Diameter is classified as Small, Normal or Large. The test to determine diameter is relatively simple. Compare a strand of your own hair to a piece of regular sewing thread.

- Thinner than thread   = small diameter
- Same thickness as thread = normal diameter
- Larger than thread   = large diameter

People who define their hair as "fine" generally have small diameter hair. The challenge for fine diameter (and low density) is to find lightweight products that will not weigh the hair down thus decreasing hair volume. Those with large diameter (and high density) strands are often seeking heavier weight products to help control hair's bulk. Turn to Chapter 7 to record your diameter rating for future use in your Customized Hair Health Plan.

DENSITY

Density is the number of active hair follicles per square inch. Don't worry, I won't ask you to count individual hairs!

To determine density:

<u>For longer hair:</u>

Step 1: pull hair back into a firmly secured ponytail using a soft fabric band without metal closures.

Step 2: Compare the size of the hair bundle as follows:

- Size of a dime – low density
- Size of a quarter – medium density
- Size of a half-dollar coin – high density

<u>For shorter hair:</u>

Hold a section of hair firmly and gently hold the section tautly away from the scalp

- Low density – generally scalp can be seen through the section of hair
- Medium density – it is harder to see the scalp in the section of hair
- High Density – it is relatively difficult to see the scalp within the section of hair being held

Unfortunately, you can't increase the number of follicles or permanently increase the diameter of the hair, so why do you need to know these characteristics?

1. Chemical processing time and product strength vary. For example, my hair is Fine Diameter, High Density, Very Curly hair. During the years I attempted to wear relaxed hair, it would end up overprocessed because the stylists would call that "coarse hair." They would use a higher strength product. Instead, this hair type would indicate a milder strength product, but the need to work quickly to apply through high density hair. Processing time should have been below or at the recommended processing time.

2. If you experience diffuse hair loss, knowing your norm helps you determine progress in regrowth. Diffuse loss occurs when there aren't bald spots but there is more hair loss than normal occurring

evenly throughout the scalp.

One last thing to note, large diameter hair doesn't indicate "coarse" hair. More often than not, coarseness is based on the condition of the cuticle.

Now, turn to Chapter 7 to record your density rating.

ELASTICITY

Elasticity is the ability of a strand of hair to stretch and return to its original length without breaking. Healthy hair should be able to stretch up to 50% of its length and return to normal. For example, a 3 inch strand of hair should be able to be stretched to 4.5 inches and return to 3 inches when no longer stretched.

Elasticity is a vital part of hair health because it measures the strength of the cross-bonds (disulfide bonds) within the hair strand. Virgin (unprocessed) hair in good condition should be highly elastic. Hair that has been bleached, permanently colored, permed, or relaxed has had the cross bonds broken and reformed. Based on the condition of the hair prior to service, the skill of the stylist performing the service, and how long chemicals are left to process in the hair, some of the bonding in the hair may never reform because the disulfide, also known as cystine, bond had been converted to cysteic acid. This reaction is irreversible.

How do you test your hair's elasticity?
1. Lay a dry strand of hair on the table with one end taped down
2. Use a ruler or tape measure to measure the stand when pulled just enough to be straight. (ex.3 inches)
3. Use half of the measurement taken in step 2. (ex.1.5 inches)
4. Pull the strand until it reaches the total distance in steps 2 & 3 (3+1.5=4.5 inches)
5. Release the tension on the strand and look at the

strand for any signs of distortion (ex. splitting, breakage, thinner areas along the length of the strand).

If you see signs of breakage or distortion, the elasticity is poor. If you have poor elasticity, you are at high risk for damage and breakage during chemical services. You should limit chemical services to preserve your hair.

What should you do about poor elasticity?

I would suggest a deep conditioning using a product with higher percentages of protein. This will not replace the disulfide bonds that were destroyed, but it will help save the hair as you continue to grow out new, healthy hair.

Turn to Chapter 7 to record your elasticity rating.

CURL PATTERN

I bet I know what you are thinking. We aren't going to be "typing" our hair using alphabets and numbers. We will also absolutely not be judging hair as "good" or "bad." Let's discuss straightness, waviness and curliness.

The origin of texture is generally believed to be the shape of the follicle. Perfectly round follicles grow straight hair. The more oval or flattened the follicle, the greater the degree of curl or wave.

One point to note is that major changes in the sex hormones (puberty, pregnancy, post-childbirth, menopause, hysterectomy, etc.) can cause texture changes. For that reason, I caution against chemical processing for children under age 12.

All that being said, let's get back to texture and its

role in healthy hair. Straight hair is characterized as hair with no discernable wave pattern. That doesn't mean there isn't frizz. Remember, porosity is a major factor in hair's response to humidity. In straight hair, sebum (oil from the scalp) is most easily distributed. When the cuticle is not damaged, straight hair often looks shiny since light has an even surface to reflect light.

Wavy hair is characterized by a distinct pattern of bends in the hair. Whether the bend is every 2 inches or every 1 centimeter, hair can still be classified as wavy.

In contrast, curly hair often coils, which we're defining as a sharp change in the direction of hair growth. Curly and wavy hair aren't entirely different since some people have tight curls until their hair reaches longer lengths. Often, the hair then appears to have a wave pattern. This is due to the weight of the stand preventing the hair from "coiling" into a tight pattern. Once the length is cut off, the remaining shorter hair may well then display the coiled effect.

So what about kinky hair? First, the term has negative connotations. It is often used interchangeably with "nappy," which indicates hair is in an undesirable state. Also, upon close inspection, even the tightest coil has a pattern. If the stand is stretched slightly, it will become apparent that there is a regular alternation of bends in the hair. When the hair reaches a longer length, the pattern is often more easily seen.

So, what distinguishes curly and wavy hair? Many find that the smaller the curl, the more susceptible the hair is to dryness and frizz. Remember the cuticle has lifting at the point where the hair growth changes direction. This often contributes to higher porosity, more dryness, and frizz. The distinction between these types has more to do with the amount of detangling, conditioning and moisturizing needed as well as finding the right weight of product for those specific needs.

Let's briefly review the highlights of each type of curl pattern:

- Straight hair – the challenge is to avoid cuticle damage. Gentle hair brushing, limiting heat application and conditioning are key.

- Wavy Hair – the challenge is avoiding damage, perfecting the styling routine to emphasize pattern, moisturizing, and preventing tangles.

- Curly Hair – the challenge is to avoid damage, perfect the styling routine to emphasize coil pattern, detangling, moisturizing, and deep conditioning are key. Leave-in moisturizers and/or curl enhancing products are generally needed.

So what does it mean to "emphasize pattern?" Many stylists experienced in cutting wavy and curly hair have perfected a method of cutting hair at an angle just below the bend of the curl. Cutting hair in this manner helps minimize frizz, encourages ringlets (or clusters of strands), and gives hair a defined shape. In addition, a stylist experienced in cutting wavy/curly hair may help you build or reduce volume using the texture of your hair.

The chart briefly summarizes key differences between the curl patterns.

Property	Straight	Wavy	Curly
Shine	Highest	Less than straight	Least amount of shine
Tangling	Least likely	More likely	Most likely
Moisture level	Varies	Tends to be drier	Tends to be dry/very dry
Frequency of cleansing/ conditioning	Most frequent – can be daily or every other day as needed	May consider every other day or every few days	May vary between every few days and weekly

If you haven't already captured your curl pattern in the Customized Healthy Hair plan, turn to chapter 7 now to do so.

CHAPTER 4
HEAT & CHEMICALS:
HOW THEY AFFECT THE HAIR

In this chapter we're going to build on your knowledge of your hair type and the state of your hair. In addition to the characteristics of your hair, generally you will fall into one or more of the following categories:

1) Virgin, or unprocessed hair – no color, no chemicals
2) Texture altered – chemicals were used to straighten or add texture to your hair.
3) Color treated – semi-permanent, permanently colored, bleached
4) Gray

I reached out to a stylist who specializes in healthy hair care and restoration to ask what her recommended maximum temperature would be for heat styling. She replied that 350 degrees should be hot enough to style hair and safely preserve its health.

Also, be sure to note that relaxer/perm solutions are made at very high (basic pH) or very low pH (acidic). They are designed to break the bonds of the hair to be reformed into either a straight or curled pattern. The skin, while made of protein, is not nearly as resistant to chemicals as the hair can be. The chemicals from relaxers, perms, or even hair colorants/bleach coming into contact with skin for prolonged periods of time will cause chemical burns. Aside from the pain and discomfort of the burns, the scabbing, and the period of time needed to heal, this type of injury can even cause hair loss. The bottom line is if you choose to use chemicals on the hair, make sure you keep chemicals off the skin by "basing" the scalp with a petroleum jelly. Why petroleum? It forms a non-reactive, water resistant barrier that can slow the spread of the chemicals onto the skin. These chemicals tend to become more fluid once applied to hair attached to a warm scalp!

Let's begin this part of the journey with virgin hair…

1. Virgin Hair & Heat – to minimize the number of passes on sections of hair, separate hair into sections no larger than 1.5 inches by 0.5 inches when using the blowdryer, flat iron, hot comb, or the "feather flat." To further prevent damage to hair, select a good heat protectant (see Chapter 6 for product selection information).

   Virgin Hair & Chemicals – Depending on the length and density of hair, you may have an extremely difficult time altering hair texture in one session. I would caution against doing at home texture alteration on a full head of unprocessed hair. In the case of long length, high density hair, the application process would require speed and a precise application to ensure even processing throughout the hair. Don't risk ruining your beautiful hair, see a professional.

Also, the rules of chemical processing apply. Always ensure your hair has been cleansed of excessive product buildup before a chemical service. By having uniformly clean hair, you decrease the odds of uneven processing where the product buildup slowed the reaction of the chemical with the hair in some areas and processed normally in others. The end result would be hair with definite areas of damage. Most products recommend having hair dried 24-48 hours before receiving chemical services. The reason is to ensure the hydrogen and ionic bonds are intact. This only occurs when hair is dry.

2)Texture altered and/or color treated hair & heat - Remember, whenever you change the texture (perming to add curl, relaxing to remove curl) or perform permanent color or bleaching, your hair loses some of the cross linking disulfide bonds that give strength to the hair. In the case of bleaching then adding permanent color, this scenario is the most damaging of all the chemical processes.[4] Our recommended maximum temp was 350 degrees, but you should try to avoid heat whenever possible.

Hair can be pulled (gently) into a ponytail secured with fabric bands along the entire length of the ponytail. Tie hair back with a satin scarf and let the hair dry while you are asleep. When hair is dry, you may have to apply some heat to smooth out the hair or boost waves/curls. Again, make sure you apply a good heat protector before applying heat. Using ones that contain protein may extend the length of time hair stays straightened. The proteins bind to the hair shaft and help form a lightweight barrier that can help hair resist humidity.

Texture altered and/or colored hair & chemicals – the key here is to never overlap chemicals onto the previously processed hair. In order to do this you need a skilled stylist or the ability to distinguish between new growth and the older hair. For this reason, it is normally recommended that chemical services are not preformed more than every 6-8 weeks. In theory, this gives you enough time to grow enough hair to manage the new hair without overlap. Keep in mind that hair is weakest at the point where the new growth and previously processed hair meet. If performed correctly, the newly processed hair is altered to the same extent as the previously processed hair. If overlap occurs, the previously processed hair will have fewer intact disulfide bonds in the hair. This creates a weak point between sections of the hair that are not uniformly processed. Usually, the client with unevenly processed hair will see breakage over time, if not shortly after the service is complete.

Another concern is dual processing. If at all possible, avoid permanent color and/or bleaching too closely to texture altering processes. Both coloring/bleaching and texture alterations break the disulfide bonds. You are asking for a loss of elasticity each time these combinations are used on the same section of hair. Remember, loss of elasticity means hair breaks easily. This may not be an issue for those maintaining ultra short hair. Successfully accumulating substantial length with dual processes will be the exception, not the rule, and incredibly difficult to maintain.

3)Colored treated/bleached –
There are many ways to enhance the color of your hair. We will cover some of the more popular varieties.
Semi-permanent colors use chemicals that largely coat the cuticle and will last through several shampoos. These are the least damaging of the commercial types. Using color safe shampoos will help maximize the time you retain the semi-permanent color.
Permanent colorants actually perform their reaction and deposit the color particles within the cortex of the hair which make this a "permanent" color. Care must be taken to use products, particularly cleansers, that don't strip hair. So if you have permanent color, avoid "clarifying" shampoos and sulfate cleansing systems. Sulfates are such "aggressive" cleansers that they can strip color that has

been added to the hair.

Bleaching the hair typically constitutes the use of peroxide to remove the natural color from the hair. After color is removed, clients usually then have a permanent color applied. Of all the chemical processes received, this combination is the most damaging. If you choose to bleach/color, be diligent about your conditioning. Be gentle with your hair by minimizing heat, keeping hair free of split ends, and moisturizing as needed.

4)Gray hair & heat

First, it's important to note that gray hair is hair in which the melanocytes (pigment producing cells) did not infuse pigment into the hair cells as they migrate into position to form the hair strand. The hairs themselves are technically white. Some report gray hair as "more coarse" than their previously pigmented hair. The onset of gray often coincides with a hormonal change that may change the texture of your hair. During this change, the diameter may change, the curl pattern could be elongated (likely not to make hair feel coarse) or shorter causing cuticle lifting (which can make hair feel less smooth than in the past.) Regardless, it is a good idea to go back through your Customized Hair Health plan any time you have a significant change in your hair.

Heat is, however, a significant concern. People with gray hair will want to use the least possible amount of heat. Overheating the hair may cause scorching and discoloration of the hair. You have probably seen people with yellowish or brown sections in their gray hair. As recommended for the other groups, always use heat protection as well. Keep the heat to a minimum temperature and keep the tool moving through the hair. Letting a hot iron sit in the hair too long can have the same scorching affect.

Gray Hair & Chemicals – Depending on the porosity and

diameter of the new gray hair, you may find that the chemical processing timing may be different. For example, a decrease in porosity and a cuticle in better condition than the old hair from that follicle may suggest a longer processing time.

Now, let's look at the chemical processes in detail.

RELAXERS AND TEXTURIZERS:

Relaxers are products that use a high pH cream to break the disulfide bonds in the hair. These are the strongest bonds in the hair and in order to establish a new curl pattern (or lack thereof), they must be broken and reformed. Although these products have been sold for years in a do-it-yourself kit, this is one of the most damaging chemical processes that can be done to your hair, so they take a great amount of skill to do correctly. Also, the re-application process must be done correctly to prevent points of uneven processing along the hair shaft which are prone to weakness and ultimately leads to breakage. For these reasons, I recommend leaving this type of processing to the professionals.

Relaxers work by using the pH to break the bonds, but the reconfiguration is done during the smoothing step. Once the hair is completely coated with the relaxer, the next step involves smoothing the hair straight. If you remember our discussion about skin and hair differences, you'll remember that while hair can withstand these high pH levels, skin cannot. So it is vital to keep the product off of the ears, neck, forehead, and scalp during this process. For this reason, many stylists "base" the scalp using a petroleum based crème to shield those areas from the relaxer. Because you may have different curl patterns throughout your hair, your stylist should always perform a consultation to evaluate your hair and discuss your previous relaxer experiences before beginning. This information helps the stylist determine the strength of product needed, which section to begin, and how long the relaxer should remain on the hair. He or she should also be discussing the desired level of straightness you desire.

If you simply want a looser curl or wave, texturizing is the process of leaving the relaxer on for a shorter period of time, thus preventing the complete straightening of the hair. There are also formulas marketed as texturizers that use a weaker formula than a regular relaxer and give the stylist more processing time. The result is usually a looser curl or wave. You may also read about texlaxing on the internet. This is a modification to a relaxer by coating the hair with oil or adding oil to the relaxer crème. The end goal is to dilute the relaxer effect. One thing to note, the relaxing process is a precise process that needs to be duplicated every time you get a touch-up service, varying the strength of the relaxer or timing is a recipe for inconsistent processing, damage, and eventually breakage or loss of hair.

The next step in relaxing/texturizing is neutralizing. Every bit of the relaxer is rinsed from the hair, then the neutralizing shampoo is applied. This step uses a very low pH shampoo to cause the bonds to reform and stops the action of the relaxer. Some brands advocate conditioning before neutralizing. Remember, conditioners use fatty alcohols and other large molecule ingredients to bond to the hair. You want the disulfide bonds to reform with no interference so that the strength of your hair will be restored. Anything that may hinder the bond reformation is damaging your hair. Therefore, I recommend not conditioning before neutralizing.

Once the hair is completely neutralized, slather on all the conditioners you like. Sit under the dryer, if desired, then rinse them out and proceed with styling.

So what kind of ingredients are used in relaxers? Sodium hydroxide, calcium hydroxide, guanidine carbonate, guanidine hydroxide, thioglycolic acid, lithium hydroxide are some of the more popular ingredients.

So what should each hair type remember...

Highly porous hair will process more quickly, so the strength of product should be mild or regular, super is usually too strong. Low porosity hair may take a bit longer to process, the stylist should address whether to use regular or super strength and the amount of time needed based on that choice.

Low elasticity hair types should avoid the relaxing process until a series of deep conditioning treatments help restore strength to the hair. Only after hair shows an improvement in elasticity, should you consider getting a relaxer. Not heeding this advice may lead to hair that starts to break during or within days of receiving a relaxer.

It is important to note that many people relax their hair at home or with a stylist and have healthy, beautiful hair. However, there are many more who end up with brittle, lifeless hair with substantial amounts of breakage. If you find yourself in the second category, please find a stylist to help you correct this or consider giving up the relaxer process altogether.

PERMANENT WAVES (PERMS):

This product type refers to a method of breaking the disulfide bonds in the hair to reform them with a wave or curl pattern (usually done on straight hair). The size of the curl is determined by the size roller selected, and the direction of the curl is determined in the way the rollers are wound. Forget the frizzy, bushy perms of the 1980s, many advances in perm solutions, application techniques, and products to control frizz have made perming much more advanced than in the past. Today, there are many types of perms on the market.

Acid perms often use three products: activator, waving solution, and neutralizer with the addition of heat to fuel the chemical process. Many stylists will avoid this perm type because it can contain glyceryl monothioglycolate which can induce allergic reactions in sensitive clients. However, in many salons the acid perm is still used because it is deemed milder than many other types. For those with high porosity hair, it might be a good choice since it processes more slowly.

Exothermic wave solutions work more quickly because the formula creates the heat that speeds up processing. This perm type may be better suited for those with low porosity (or describe their hair as "resistant" to chemical processing. The pH is high in these perms and they often release unpleasant ammonia gas.

Endothermic perm systems require the addition of heat to work. They are similar to acid perms but are formulated to perform at different pH levels. For those with low elasticity, small diameter, and low density many stylists opt for lower pH solutions. While the outcome is usually not a well-defined curl, these solutions can produce nice wave patterns.

Thio-free waves use compounds like cysteamine or mercaptamine as a substitute for thioglycolate based systems. Be aware they can still damage hair and the curl will not be as tightly formed as the thioglycolate systems.

The bottom line to consider is that perming is chemical processing. Choosing the right formula for your hair type can be daunting and the right technique can be a challenge. So for the safest, most beautiful curl, wave, or root lift choose a stylist who specializes in these processes. Again, make sure he or she does a pre-service consultation to understand your hair type and what result you desire.

KERATIN/AMINO ACID/
TEMPORARY STRAIGHTENING:

This is the hottest, most rapidly changing product/process segment in recent history. Here we will cover the most popular types and what you need to know about them.

The Japanese Hair Straightening System® is a permanent hair straightener. It uses the thioglycolate compounds like perms except all steps require the hair to be kept in a straightened form so that the result is straight hair. The general process used is as follows:

1) Hair is completely saturated with the thioglycolate solution then after a period, rinsed, blow dried, then flatironed with high heat.

2) Next, the neutralizer is applied, hair is rinsed, dried again then flatironed again.

Given the number of times the hair is wet, then dried, the process can take 4 hours or more (depending on density and length of hair). Most systems required the hair be kept as straight as possible for 3 days. Clients will have to return for touch-ups on the new growth. Those with previously relaxed hair should know that this process is not compatible with the previously relaxed hair if hydroxide type relaxers were used..

Next, we have the Brazilian Keratin treatment®. It differs from the Japanese straightener in that it isn't formulated to be permanent. There was a fair amount of controversy associated with this method, as the original version contained relatively high levels of formaldehyde. Therefore, there was a significant health risk from inhaling formaldehyde for both the stylist and the client. This issue was hot enough for the Food and Drug Administration (FDA) to publish guidance to manufacturers and warnings to stylists and clients.

Manufacturers must keep the emission of formaldehyde at a very low level. Formaldehyde may be a listed ingredient or can be emitted by compounds such as formalin, octyl aldehyde, methylene glycol, methanediol, formic aldehyde, methyl aldehyde and other substances. So be aware of the risk and talk through this with the stylist to ensure she or he has chosen the safest product and cautionary measures so neither of you are exposed unnecessarily. According to the FDA, signs of exposure include "eye/nose irritation, headaches, dizziness, respiratory issues, nausea, chest pain, vomiting and rash." If you experience any of these symptoms during services, the FDA encourages you to contact them for further investigation.

The process varies widely by product but follows the same general process:

1) Hair is shampooed to remove all styling product and debris from the hair. These products rely on the ability of the active ingredients to bond with the hair and buildup prevents even processing. No conditioner applied here.

2) The treatment is applied to unconditioned hair. Hair is then dried then flatironed.

3) Some versions rinse, re-dry, then flatiron again

With these straightening systems, the flatiron temp is recommended to be at least 400 degrees (or higher). Remember, this temperature is above the recommended heat setting of 350 degrees. Many often suggest your maintenance hair cleanser be sulfate free and sodium chloride free. (Sodium chloride is often used as a thickener in sulfate based cleansers). This step would help decrease your odds of stripping the bonded product from the hair since the process is supposed to last for months.

The appeal of Keratin/Amino acid treatments is the promise to provide straightness that lasts through many washings but isn't supposed to be permanent. I say "supposed" because some have found that once they stop getting these treatments their natural curl pattern does not return. It is something to consider which means you may want to alternate between these processes and wearing your hair in its natural state if that is a concern for you.

Even as I write this book, there are new clay-based straighteners made from white clay from Morocco and every other exotic location imaginable. From what is disclosed by these manufacturers, this product type blends clay and protein. The steps include:

1. Washing the hair thoroughly then blow drying it.

2. Apply ¼" from the scalp, coat hair but don't oversaturate.

3.   Allow to sit on hair for 20 minutes
4.   Blow dry completely
5.   Flat iron small sections at (you guessed it) 400 degrees. Some brands advise flat-ironing the same section multiple times to ensure the desired straightness is obtained.

There are a few components of the instructions that lead me to suspect there are some ingredients not being disclosed. These indicators are "apply ¼" from the scalp, wear gloves during application". What is in these products to make these precautions necessary?

Again, the bottom line here, I never recommend being on the cutting edge of these new treatments. Anyone remember "Rio" all natural straightener? For those too young to remember, visit Wikipedia for a quick timeline and summary. I don't want to discourage you from the next big hair care breakthrough, but the science of the matter is that it takes a very low or very high pH product to break and reform the disulfide bonds in the hair. A product that can do those things wouldn't be safe to eat or smooth on your skin as a treatment as some products suggest.

While the FDA is the consumer's advocacy agency, it is not staffed or chartered to review every product that enters the market for safety, that being said, neither is Wal-Mart, Target, or the local beauty supply store. That means the consumer has to be diligent and be your own best advocate for the health and beauty of your hair.

Thermal damage is an ever growing risk as the desire to go from straight to the natural curl pattern without chemical straighteners increases. Flatirons, feather flats, blowdryers, and curling irons are in demand today with some manufacturers boasting temperatures above 450 degrees. Even with heat protectants, the hair is being scorched. For those using some heat protectants and high heat irons, the return to the original curl pattern is difficult. Extremely high heat can break the disulfide bonds in the hair, resulting in change to the curl pattern.

Currently, there are even flat irons that promise to take hair from wet-to-straight. Never apply high heat in this manner to avoid causing internal fracturing of the hair shaft as any moisture inside is literally boiled.

Blow dryers can also wreak havoc on hair if used too frequently, using high heat, and lingering (or doing many passes) over the same section of hair. Always detangle before blow drying hair. Use small sections, 0.5"x2", apply heat protectant, use the lowest heat setting possible, and maximize the amount of air (speed). If you can, try alternating between blow drying and allowing hair to air dry.

CHAPTER 5
HAIR & SCALP CONDITIONS

In reading this book, you may have noticed the term "trichologist." The term refers to the formal training and certification in the study of the hair, scalp, and conditions that affect each.

Some may call the professional a "hair doctor," but a trichologist takes a holistic look at the physical symptoms of the hair and scalp. We then use knowledge of hair, body systems, nutrition and proper hair care techniques to help clients recover from hair loss and damage.

Why not see a doctor or dermatologist instead? Many clients already have. In some cases, the dermatologist was able to diagnose and treat the condition(s). In other cases ,such as perpetual hair breakage, many clients leave the dermatologist without a plan to restore healthy hair especially when the causes are not biological.

What about seeing a stylist? Often clients start with the stylist, but many causes of hair loss or breakage aren't thoroughly incorporated into beauty school curriculums.

This is where the trichologist can effectively partner with your dermatologist, doctor, and/or stylist to help restore your hair. In this chapter, we will cover some basic hair and scalp conditions, what to look for, and the steps to take in order to remedy these conditions.

HAIR BREAKAGE

Hair breakage is often described as "my hair won't grow." What's actually occurring is that the ends or strands of hair are breaking at the same rate as hair growth resulting in no gain in length. Hair breakage is usually caused by: splits in the hair shaft (trichorrhexis nodosa), Split ends (trichoptilosis), knots at the end of hair (referred to as fairy knots by some) or damage within the hair shaft.

Trichorrhexis nodosa can occur multiple times along the same strand of hair. Unfortunately, cutting the strand above the first split is the only way to rid the hair of this type of damage. In some cases, you can see this with the naked eye.

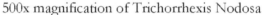

500x magnification of Trichorrhexis Nodosa

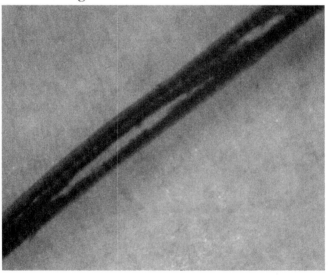

This condition is caused by poorly formed, weakened hair, mechanical, thermal, or chemical damage that erodes the cuticle. Without an intact cuticle, the exposed cortex splits in various places along the length of the hair strand.

Trichoptilosis (split ends) is caused by friction of hair against clothing, excessive wear and tear of the oldest part of the hair, dryness, and/or thermal damage. Again, trimming above the split is the only way to rid the hair of the split ends.

500x magnification of Trichoptilosis

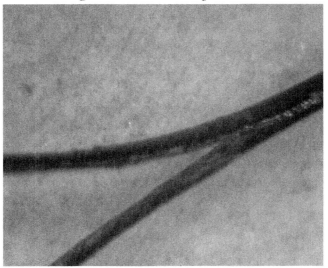

Bubble hair is damage that can only be seen under a microscope but is very real. When the strand is overheated, moisture within the strand is literally boils significantly damaging the hair. This would be one reason to never flatiron wet hair. The second reason being you may likely get a nasty steam burn. Essentially, the hair may not look outwardly different, but it feels brittle/rough to the touch. This texture indicates that the hair has been damaged and is very weak making it susceptible to further damage. Deep conditioning and moisturizing may improve the feel of the hair but unfortunately the damage is done.

What about the products that promise to mend split ends?

In order to repair a split end, the product would need to penetrate the strand, reform the disulfide (cross bonds), and rebuild any of the cuticle that is damaged. Unfortunately, products on the market today can't do that. The ones that claim to mend split ends are using polymers the temporary bind the fragments together. The problem is that the damage inside the shaft will continue to expand up the hair shaft. An analogy to consider is a pair of pantyhose/stockings with a "run". The longer you wear the hose, the worse the "run" becomes. The longer you leave the split in the hair strand, the more damage that strand will receive. In order to save the strand, be diligent about cutting the damage off when you see it.

Knots at the end of the strand (commonly referred to as fairy knots) are almost exclusively caused by friction between strands of hair or against the clothing. I would love to tell you that it's possible to "untie" each one but that's just not practical. The solution is to trim the hair just above the knot. If you don't, other hairs will often "catch" on one another and cause a larger mass of tangles.

500x magnification of a "fairy knot"

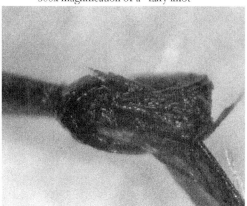

The proactive thing to do to prevent the knots is to practice protective styling. Protective styling involves 1) gently detangling the hair frequently, 2) preventing the ends from being damaged by environmental factors and friction, 3) avoiding excessive tension, and 4) moisture sealing.

1) How to detangle hair without pain and breakage:

Detangling the hair to avoid introducing knots is an art all its own. Start with small sections of hair. First, use your fingers to separate strands within the small section. If you are detangling while hair is wet, make sure you are especially gentle. The key is to start at the ends and slowly move upward. Never pull hair forcefully apart, this can cause the mechanical damage that leads to splits within the hair shaft or snap the hair immediately. Next, starting at the ends, use a wide tooth comb and work your way up towards the roots starting an inch higher, combing down, then repeating. **Every time** the comb catches a mass of hair that tangles, immediately stop and separate the hair with your fingers. If you don't, by the time you reach the ends, you will have a massive knot of hair. To make detangling easier, apply a moisturizer with a pH between

4.5-5.5. In that range, the cuticle lies flatly and makes hairs less likely to "catch" on each other.

2)Preventing ends from rubbing against clothing, etc.

To prevent damage to your ends, think of styles that help keep ends from being exposed. Examples would include buns, updos, etc. I know everyone likes variety in styling, but tucking your ends away on occasion, the more often the better, reduces the friction, limits exposure to sun and air, and helps keep ends moisturized. Some opt for total rest for the hair using wigs and extensions. These are perfectly viable options provided they are done correctly.

Let's begin with wigs. Full wigs can allow damaged hair a complete retreat from daily styling and exposure to the environment. However, there are a few practices that will help you achieve your protective goals. Wear a wig cap. There are several kinds on the market and most often you will see the "stocking" kind. Many women avoid this type, especially if they sweat on the scalp or get hot very easily. By the way, one of the earliest indicators of Vitamin D deficiency was excessive sweating of the scalp. (See a doctor for blood testing if you suspect this might hold true for you.) A cooler wig cap option is the "net" type that has holes between the weaving that allow for better circulation of air. Either way, a cap is essential for 2 reasons: to prevent breakage of the fragile hair around the hairline and to minimize friction between the wig and the rest of your hair. Also, if you opt for a wig, you MUST continue to cleanse, condition, moisturize, and detangle your own hair. If you don't, expect breakage, sweaty/itchy scalp, and perhaps scalp flaking.

Weaving hair can also provide protection, if done correctly and proper care of the natural hair is done regularly. First with weaving, your hair is usually braided and used as a base for attachment of tracks. Before you put your hair "away," make sure it has been effectively cleansed, conditioned, moisturized, and detangled. Ensure your stylist does not braid so tightly that you have pain.

Protecting hair at night is really an extension of previous advice. Allowing hair to remain loose during sleep is an excellent way to tangle, dry hair out and break it. Instead, simply detangle hair as detailed earlier in the chapter, moisturize if needed, and separate into loose braids or twists. Some prefer to wrap hair around the head to maintain straightness. One word of caution here, be careful not to apply too much tension from the wrapping or the pins used to secure ends. The excessive tension can cause pain and inflammation to the follicles. Next, either sleep in a satin cap or on a satin pillowcase, by doing so you will prevent excessive friction between the hair and linens. Also, moisture from the hair is absorbed by cotton sheets or pillowcases if a satin barrier isn't used.

3)Pain indicates stress on the follicle.

If the braid is painful, attaching the hair will only intensify the stress. Weaves are generally attached in one of three ways: gluing, sewing, or clips. With glue, many people learn after the application that they have an allergic response to the glue (itching, burning, etc.) For that reason, glue is best patch tested on skin before you have an expensive weave completed that must be removed. Also, know that it must be removed very carefully to avoid plucking or breaking the attached hair.

When considering sewing, know that any extension attached to hair that is pulled to begin the braid, is likely to cause breakage (or loss) of that hair. Sewing attached to the braid uses the braided bundle of hair whereas the unbraided hair that starts the braid is already under tension of the braid. Adding the tension of the weaving thread and weight of the extensions can cause trauma to follicles. The rest of the braided hair is also at risk for damage if the weaving thread is too tight.

Finally, using clips to hold in extensions can be a less damaging process, as long as you use the "pain" test. None of these styling methods should hurt.

One final note on extensions. I see many young girls/women with waist length extensions or braids. Often the extension/braid texture is very different from their own hair type causing "edge control" to be a major styling issue. The edge control industry is a booming business using heavy ingredients to essentially "glue" the hair down under high tension or with extensive brushing. Add this to the weight of the extensions and the tension of the braided natural hair, and many finish their weave period with broken or no edge hair due to traction alopecia (loss of hair due to high tension). Sadly, many continue these practices until the hairline is permanently damaged and the hair will never grow back (cicatricial alopecia).
1) Moisture Sealing – (see technique on page 18)
Hair that is allowed to become dry is brittle and prone to damage. Be diligent in keeping your hair moisturized.

HAIR LOSS
This is an area where you should learn to recognize the signs, then proceed to a professional as soon as possible. Hair loss is one of the body's indicators that there is an issue. As a practicing trichologist, I see clients with a variety of hair loss conditions. We will discuss some of the most common conditions.

Diffuse hair loss is loss of hair throughout the scalp, not isolated to a spot of baldness. Those experiencing it notice their hair is "not as full as it used to be."

Diffuse loss is a decrease in density of hair. Some notice the ponytail isn't as thick as it once was where others can see more scalp that they normally can.

In almost all cases the cause is internal. The causes vary from nutritional deficiency, medical condition onset, adverse reaction to medication, or even a shock to the body system. Because there are such wide ranges of cause, a professional is needed to help you address the root cause and get on the path to restoring your hair. This is the role of a certified trichologist who may, in turn, refer you to your medical doctor for confirmation and treatment.

Hair loss that occurs in defined patches is clinically called alopecia (partial or complete absence of hair). The specific pattern of loss is how the different types of alopecia are diagnosed. Alopecia areata is a specific area of hair loss. This condition is generally an autoimmune issue, where the body attacks its own cells, in this case hair cells resulting in hair loss.

Hair loss in a specific area can also be the aftermath of an area that was affected by chemical burns or heavy scaling. Once the scab or scaling is removed, the hair comes out leaving an area of baldness. In these instances, run, don't walk to see a trichologist who can help identify the cause and help you restore as much hair as possible. Depending on the cause, early diagnosis and treatment may help prevent the spread of the affected area.

Trichologists also often see androgentic alopecia. This type of loss causes male pattern baldness in men but is becoming more and more common in women. This type of loss is "genetic" and fueled by the effects of androgens on the hair follicle. Typically in men, there's a receding hairline that may continue until the entire front and top are bald, leaving hair actively growing over the ears and around to the nape of the neck. In women, the same area may be affected but usually to a lesser extent. There are a variety of treatment options available and it's better to address the loss as soon as possible rather than later.

In Chapter 1, we covered the inner root sheath and its role in helping to hold a growing hair in the follicle. Loose anagen syndrome is a disorder that causes loss of a growing hair due to weakness of the connective tissue (the inner root sheath). Once the condition is properly diagnosed, there are treatment plans to help restore the strength of the inner root sheath. This condition mostly occurs in females with light colored hair but can be seen in other hair colors and types as well.

When illnesses cause hair loss it is usually diffuse hair loss. Nutritional deficiency, digestive issues (that cause malabsorption of nutrients), thyroid, diabetes, lupus, psoriasis, and many other health conditions can cause hair loss. The reason the trichological consultation is so effective is that we look for such triggers and help develop a treatment plan for you.

SCALP CONDITIONS
One of the most common scalp symptoms is pruritis, or itching of the scalp. Excessive itch can be caused by many conditions, we'll cover a few of the most common.
Dandruff (Pityriasis Capitis) – small, white flakes that form on the scalp. Dandruff is annoying but generally harmless. It is believed to be caused by yeast overgrowth of the scalp. The scalp attempts to rid itself of the excess yeast growth by producing and shedding skin cells at a higher than normal rate. Dandruff is treated with an ingredient like selenium sulfide, zinc pyrithione, or ketoconazole which acts on the yeast to

control their growth and return the natural balance to the scalp. Other formulas use salicylic acid to help the scalp shed the top layers of skin and yeast in the process.

Another cause of itchy scalp can simply be dryness. If this is the cause, applying a pre-shampoo treatment containing a high percentage of aloe vera and an oil that that quickly absorbs into the skin (like coconut oil or almond oil). This can help give your scalp the moisture and oil that it may be missing. Pre-treating the scalp can be even more beneficial if you gently massage the scalp using the pads of your fingers. Never use your fingernails as that may cause broken skin and lead to serious infections.

Itchy scalp may also be caused by allergic reactions to products used on the hair. Many people find that they experience itching after coloring the hair. If you notice this, take note of the brand of colorant and the ingredients used. Ask your colorist to use a different color system or choose another brand if you are coloring at home. The next time you encounter this colorant, you may be faced with a full-blown allergic reaction. To soothe the itch from a possible pre-allergic response, wash the hair with a shampoo you have not had reaction issues with the past. Make sure to thoroughly massage the entire scalp and rinse thoroughly to remove any potential product residue that may have been left on the scalp.

If you find that you have itching and yellow flakes or scales (large flakes, often still attached to the scalp), you're dealing with conditions much more complicated that dandruff. In the case of large, yellowish flakes that cling to the hair, this may be dermatitis. Large scales stuck to the scalp may be a variety of conditions such as psoriasis, pityriasis amianticea, or other conditions. You will need a professional diagnosis. One thing to note is that you must never attempt to remove the scales still attached to the scalp or causing hair to matte to the scalp. Doing this will likely cause you to lose the hair underneath resulting in a bald spot.

Hair loss or severe scalp issues can be devastating. Beginning with the right analysis, putting treatment plan in place, and committing to alter any practices that aggravate loss can help many restore damaged or lost hair to a more healthy state.

Turn to chapter 7 to record your observations in the Customized Hair Health Plan.

CHAPTER 6
INGREDIENTS AND PRODUCT SELECTION

The hair care industry is one of the largest segments n the beauty industry. Fueled by the success stories of women who started blending products in their kitchens, new product companies emerge all the time. This fiercely competitive market gives the consumer endless options, but can also drown people in marketing misinformation.

As a chemist, my company creates products for businesses across the country under their own brand names (called private label manufacturing). The information I am about to share is the basis behind how all those products are formulated. My goal is to inform you, the consumer, so you can make educated buying decisions. Let's start with the regulatory aspect of products.

PRODUCT CATEGORIES AND CLAIMS

Cosmetics are defined as "articles intended to be rubbed, poured, sprinkled, or sprayed on, introduced into or otherwise applied to the human body...for cleansing, beautifying, promoting attractiveness or altering the appearance." FD&C Act, Section 201 (i). Drugs are defined as "articles intended for use in diagnosis, cure, mitigation, treatment or prevention of disease" and "articles (other than food) intended to affect the structure or any function of the body of man or other animals."

Cosmeceutical is a term you may hear today but it is not recognized by the FDA (Food and Drug Administration); however, a product can be classified as both a drug and a cosmetic. For example, dandruff shampoos claim to treat dandruff (drug) and cleanse hair (cosmetic).

Why is this important to you? It's important because products that claim to "grow hair" but aren't classified as drugs are either misleading you or are mislabeled. Many products help minimize breakage but that isn't the same as causing hair to grow. The concern is that a company should never mislead the consumer.

So, to advocate for clarity for the consumer, the FDA regulates the labeling and product claims of cosmetics and drugs. Drug products have to have documentation of the studies they have done to ensure effectiveness of the product, for the claims being made, and for the safety of such products.

For cosmetics, ingredients must be listed in descending order of concentration. Translation, the first ingredient listed makes up the majority of the product. The last ingredient is the smallest amount of the product. Perhaps you already knew that, but here's an insider tip. Most preservatives make up 1% or less of the product. Anything less than that is not likely to have a noticeable effect in the product. There are a very few exceptions to that fact.

Now that we have a bit of background, let's get to the types of ingredients!

Butters: non-polar emollients from plant sources
  Examples: shea, mango, cocoa: note – some "butters" are oil extracts blended in coconut oil which is semi-solid at 76 degrees (i.e. aloe butter)

Cleansers: (also known as surfactants) remove oil and debris
  Examples: sodium lauryl sulfate, ammonium lauryl sulfate, cocamide DEA, cocamidopropyl betaine, decyl glucoside

---

Conditioners: aid in strengthening the hair and smoothing the cuticle
  Examples: behentrimonium chloride, guar hydroxypropyl trimonium chloride, hydroxypropyl trimonium honey, centrimonium chloride, polyquaternium 7,10, etc. hydrolyzed wheat protein, silk amino acids, keratin

---

Emollients: oil-based or oil-soluble substances that add gloss to the hair and aid in preventing loss or absorption of moisture
  Examples: oils, butters, waxes

Emulsifiers/thickeners: allow water based and oil based ingredients to blend together and create solutions or crèmes. Some of these same ingredients often make products thicker.
  Examples: emulsifying wax is a class of products using fatty acids and polysorbates in combination, stearic acid, xanthan gum, lecithin

---

Fatty Alcohols: used to help soften hair, thicken products and improve feel of skin or hair. They are non-drying. Examples: cetyl alcohol, cetearyl alcohol, stearyl alcohol

---

Film formers: create films used to enhance volume or hold styles
Examples: PVP, carbomer, sodium carbomer, PVM/M Copolymer

Humectants: attract and bind water.
Examples: glycerin, hyalauronic acid, sorbitol, sodium PCA, aloe vera, propylene glycol

---

Oils: non-polar substances derived from plants or petroleum
Examples: plant based – castor oil, avocado, argan, coconut, ; non-plant based – mineral oil

---

pH adjusters: used to get the product pH to 4.5-5.5, used to raise pH to help gel formation, or for perm & relaxer processing
Examples: citric acid, lactic Acid, sodium hydroxide, sodium bicarbonate

---

Preservatives: prevent growth of mold, fungi and bacteria
Examples: methyl-, propyl-, butyl-, isobutyl- parabens; grapefruit seed extract, phenoxyethanol, caprylyl glycol

---

Silicones: any of a type of synthetic materials considered polymers made of chains of alternating silicon and oxygen atoms, with organic groups attached to the silicon atoms. They are typically resistant to temperature changes and often used in heat protecting products.
Examples: dimethi-, cyclomethi-, amodimethicone

Waxes: plant based, non-polar substances that are solids at room temperature – soy, candelilla, carnauba; animal based – beeswax; Mineral based – ozokerite, ceresin, paraffin, microcrystalline

---

ANATOMY OF HAIR PRODUCTS

Now that you have an understanding of labeling and some common ingredients, let's take a closer look at some of the product forms on the market today.

CLEANSERS/SHAMPOOS:

Today there are traditional shampoos, a few 2-N-1s, conditioning cleansers and co-washes. A traditional shampoo uses a combination of surfactants that create thick, dense foam. Either they "Clarify" (or strip excess oil and debris from hair) or they promise not to strip hair of its moisture. Almost without exception, shampoos give the rich foam that consumers perceive as necessary to get the hair clean. In fact, the more foam you get, the more drying the product usually is to the hair. In most cases, it takes a combination of sulfates and secondary cleansers to get the dense foam. Also, the more oil-based ingredients you have, the less foam you have. This means that often the high foamers lack many conditioning agents which are usually oil based because the foam level is the goal. For those with dry hair (high porosity, wavy, curly hair), be aware that these products are stripping the small amount of moisture you have from your hair. In particular, sulfates are the most powerful cleansers and they also strip color from the hair.

2-N-1s are the old school attempt to combine cleansing and conditioning into one product. They still tend to use powerful surfactants to get the rich foam but may contain slightly more conditioning agents than the traditional shampoo. Again, for those hair types prone to dryness, this product will likely be too drying and not offer enough conditioning power for your hair.

Conditioning cleansers are relatively new, but the concept is to use very mild cleansers at lower percentages and to load the product with conditioning agents. The net effect is very little foam but all the benefits of a conditioner. Because there are surfactants in the product, this type of cleanser can be used on a regular basis. It's gentle enough for color-treated, dry, or damaged hair. However, It may be too heavy for the small diameter/low density type.

Finally, there's the Co-Wash. This product is marketed to those who follow the practice of using only the conditioner to cleanse the hair. The concept here is that oil can dissolve oil, so there may be no surfactants at all in certain brands. What you will find is tons of fatty acids, conditioning agents and oils/butters. It can be great for those with damaged or dry hair, however, a clarifying shampoo will be needed periodically to remove potential buildup on the hair. Think of it this way, if you only took baths using lotion, your skin would be soft and smooth, but you would still need soap to remove build-up. For those with small diameter/low density hair types, the co-wash may be too heavy for you.

The benefits of the conditioning cleanser and the co-wash are that the hair is immersed in moisture and emollient rich blends that help detangle, moisturize and can help strengthen the hair. Again, you may need to periodically use a clarifying shampoo to remove buildup from the hair.

Before we leave cleansers, let's stop to discuss the ACV movement. If you follow the blogs or social media, you will find a legion of fans. Call me a product snob, but ACV is just too harsh to use on the hair. The pH is too low, it can strip the hair, and cause it to feel brittle. Today, there are too many excellent products on the market using the correct pH balance to use ACV. In addition, mashed bananas, avocados, raw eggs, etc. are great ingredients for your recipes, but aren't nearly as effective in adding moisture, emollience, and protein as today's products. Besides, they will make for a horrible experience if you can't get the pulp and residue out of your hair.

So how should you choose a cleanser?

Most hair types should avoid sulfate based cleansers – unless you have engine oil in your hair since sulfates were originally developed as engine degreasers. For the rest of us, sulfate-free will work just fine. Look for humectants, fatty acids and emollients. As far as the pH, very few products list the pH, but an ingredients list including citric acid or lactic acid means the manufacturer was trying to lower the pH. Most conditioning agents today work at lower pH levels, so a product loaded with conditioning agents will likely be close to the right pH. If you choose to use a cleanser with sulfates, know that ammonium lauryl sulfate must be kept near neutral (pH 7) or in the acid range, so the pH is likely to be closer to the ideal range.

CONDITIONERS:

The basic job of a conditioner is to restore any moisture loss, detangle and help smooth the cuticle. To qualify as a treatment, ingredients that bond to the hair are often used. Keratin, hydrolyzed wheat protein, and silk amino acids are a few of the more common ingredients which have a positive charge that is attracted to the negative charge of damaged areas of the hair. These ingredients, used in meaningful amounts, can help fortify hair. Deep conditioners or protein treatments, etc. should not be left on the hair. If you do, hair will dry in clumps, may be hard or stiff, and you are likely to cause breakage if you comb through the hair. Here's what to look for in a conditioner.

Cetearyl alcohol (or any of the fatty alcohols) and other

conditioning agents listed in the section above, along with natural oils and butters, glycerin or other humectants. The pH of this product should be between 4.5-5.5, but many conditioning ingredients have a lower pH, so you may not see a pH adjuster listed. Low density/small diameter may want to find a lighter weight conditioner. Poor elasticity, high density, large diameter, curly, or wavy hair will probably want a thick, rich version usually in a jar or bottle with a pump.

LEAVE-IN CONDITIONERS or MOISTURIZERS:

The difference in the leave-in vs. traditional conditioner is generally the percentage and type of conditioning ingredients used. Usually, the leave-in conditioner will use lighter weight conditioning agents – so you may not see the behentrimonium type ingredients at all.

Instead, light weight conditioners, fatty acids, butters and emollients are preferred. You may also see a variety of herbal extracts but you will definitely see some humectants. For those looking for wave/curl enhancers, you may see some of the film formers as well.

HEAT PROTECTANTS:

Heat protectant products are a slight variation on liquid leave-in conditioners. The amount of humectants is generally much lower, but there is a higher amount of heat resistant ingredients. In some cases, proteins are used, in others, blends or silicones are added. The protectant provides a thin layer of product to the hair so that the higher heat of a blow dryer or flat iron won't burn the hair. Heat protectants can be effective but only when used with the correct heat settings and when heating small sections. Even the best heat protectant will struggle to protect hair from high heat concentrated in the same area for long periods of time. Also, remember to not over-apply this product as they are almost all water based, you can wet the hair which makes it more vulnerable to damage from elevated temperatures.

SPRITZ/HOLDING SPRAY/MOUSSE:

The purpose of these products is to help hold hair in place and/or give volume to hair. Spritz products are usually a thin liquid containing alcohol applied with a sprayer. The alcohol used is as a solvent for the other ingredients and a lot of the alcohol drops will not reach the hair when sprayed from the recommended distance of 8-10 inches from the hair. This can be still be drying to the hair and overuse can make the hair stiff or sticky.

Holding spray is usually in a pressurized aerosol can. The ingredients are very much like those found in spritzes with propellants added to help with the dispensing from the can. In fact, spritzes are an environmentally friendly alternative to aerosol products.

Mousse is usually in a can with a lever that dispenses foam through a tube. They usually contain water, some will have alcohol, but most will have film foamers and cleansers/surfactants to build the foam characteristics of this product type. Mousse may be used on most hair types.

SHINE SPRAYS / DROPS:

These are designed to add that sometimes elusive shine that makes hair so much more noticeable. The earliest sprays/drops used silicones. The difference in form (drop/spray) is the molecular weight of the type of silicone used. Some sprays used cyclomethicone to get the lightest weight products.

Today we are starting to see the emergence of natural oils or natural oil blends to enhance the shine of the hair. Castor oil is arguably the best natural shine enhancer but it is also very viscous or heavy on the hair. For the curly/wavy crowd, some are using pure castor oil or blends of castor/coconut oil, which is more readily absorbed into the hair.

In case, you are waiting for me to disapprove of the use of silicones, I don't plan to. Silicones form a lasting shine that is more difficult for natural oils to duplicate. However, I always advocate using natural ingredients if you can achieve the results you desire. With shine enhancing products, choose the lightest weight product that doesn't weigh your hair down or cause the hair to be sticky.

Having great shine today but having to wash your hair more frequently will prove to be more detrimental to your hair in the long run.

GELS:

This product form seems to come in go in terms of popularity. Do you remember curl activator gel? Gels make use of a film former that also thickens. They use carbomers and other variations. Next, all humectants are added to the blend and the gel is complete.

Gels that contain high levels of glycerin can leave a "wet" feel to the hair (ex. curl activator gel). Those without humectants or with small amounts of humectants can give hair a stiffer feel. Fortunately, manufacturers help you choose the right formula by providing a "hold scale" from 1 to 10 or using words to describe the hold level. Gels will almost always be too heavy for small diameter, low density hair unless you are looking to slick hair down. For high porosity, high density, wavy or curly hair, gels can be helpful when used in moderation.

POMADES/STYLING WAX/EDGE CONTROL:

Although the product names are sometimes used interchangeably, they are distinctly different product forms. First, a pomade is generally made with waxes or oils blended to achieve a very thick consistency. This product type used the weight of the ingredients to hold the hair in the desired position. For this reason, small diameter, low density hair may find that this product is way too heavy for their hair. Pomades usually work best on large diameter, high density, curly or wavy types looking for hair control during braiding, twisting, or other styling. Depending on the ingredients used (petrolatum, beeswax, microcrystalline wax), pomades can require a clarifying shampoo in order to remove the products during the cleansing process.

Styling wax is often thinner than pomades but designed to help create "spikes" or a "piecy" hair look with a water based formula. Ingredients like PEG-40 hydrogenated castor oil and ceteareth-25 are often blended and may include a carbomer base. This makes the styling wax much less oily than a pomade, but will still enable the user to control the hair in pieces or sections. This type of product would be much better for the small diameter/low density hair types. Many of the product names are changing, so you may see the term "pomade" being used for a styling wax. Generally, styling wax will be clear or creamy versus pomades which will be opaque due to the actual waxes used.

Last, but certainly not least, are edge control products. Many are formulated like the styling waxes with smaller amounts of humectants and emollients. They typically are clear solids that are heavy enough to hold the finer edge hair in place. Edge controls can be effective on all hair types. Please keep in mind that the hair around the edge of your hairline is generally the finest and most fragile. The edge control product itself is not detrimental to hair; however, the repeat brushing and pulling sometimes used with the edge control can add stress to the follicles and ultimately lead to hair loss in the future. Be mindful of the potential for damage so you don't look back later and wonder why your hairline is receding.

So how do you use all the information in this chapter to make informed buying decisions?

Start with your density, diameter, curl pattern and porosity. If your hair is easily weighed down, look for lightweight products: liquids, fluid creams, and sprays. For hold, you might want to choose a spray or styling wax.

For hair that needs more control – high density, large diameter, curly, or wavy – look for thicker, creamier products containing natural oils and butters. Your goal is to condition, detangle, moisturize and protect hair.

Obviously, there are no "one-size-fits-all" prescriptions, but get in the habit of reading the labels and ignoring the marketing hype.

CHAPTER 7
CREATING YOUR CUSTOMIZED HAIR HEALTH PLAN

In this chapter, you will be documenting what you have learned about your hair type and developing a plan for the changes you need to make to restore/better maintain the health and beauty of your hair.

Part 1– Better skin and hair from the inside out (Chapter 2)

Part 2 - Determining and documenting your hair type (Chapter 3)

Part 3 - Heat & chemicals and how they affect your hair (Chapter 4)

Part 4 – Hair & scalp conditions (Chapter 5)

Part 5 - Selecting products (Chapter 6)

<u>YOUR CUSTOMIZED HAIR HEALTH PLAN</u>

PART 1: Better skin and hair from the inside out – use the information from Chapter 2

Protein:

    ____ Yes, I get 3 or more servings of complete proteins daily

    ____ No, I get fewer than 3 servings of complete proteins per day

ACTION PLAN:

If no, how will I add protein to my diet?

_____

_____

_____

_____

Vitamins:

    ____ Yes, I eat the recommended daily amounts of the food groups, eat fresh fruits and vegetables

    ____ No, I don't consistently eat the recommended daily amounts of the foods in the food groups

ACTION PLAN:

If no, what foods I will add to my diet to make sure I get the vitamins needed for my health and therefore my hair health:

_____

_____

_____

_____

_____

YOUR CUSTOMIZED HAIR HEALTH PLAN
Minerals:

_____ Yes, my diet includes whole grains, eggs, rice, seafood, spinach and even seeds

_____ No, I avoid one or more of the foods listed above.

ACTION PLAN:

If no, foods (or supplements as directed by your physician) I will add to my diet to ensure I get the correct daily mineral supply:

_____
_____
_____

Water:

_____ Yes, I drink 64 ounces (or more) or pure water per day.

_____ No, I only drink water when it is used to make my soda, tea or flavored beverages.

ACTION PLAN:

If no, what steps will I commit to try in order to increase my water intake:

_____
_____
_____

Exercise:

_____ Yes, I get at least 20 minutes of exercise each day (or at least 30 minutes three times per week)

_____ No, I am inconsistent with exercise or I don't exercise at all

ACTION PLAN:

If no, what steps will I take to increase my daily physical activity:

_____
_____
_____

YOUR CUSTOMIZED HAIR HEALTH PLAN

PART 2: Documenting your hair type: use the information from Chapter 3

POROSITY:

____ High   ____Normal   ____ Low

DIAMETER:

____ Small   ____ Normal   ____ Large

DENSITY:

____ Low   ____ Normal   ____ High

ELASTICITY:

____ Poor   ____Good

CURL PATTERN:

____ Straight   ____ Wavy   ____ Curly

YOUR CUSTOMIZED HAIR HEALTH PLAN

PART 3: Heat and chemicals and how my hair is affected (Chapter 4)

___ Yes, my hair feels good. Breakage/damage/loss, or slow accumulation of length is not an issue for me

___ No, my hair either feels brittle, breaks easily, is damaged, or I have experienced some hair loss.

ACTION PLAN:

Heat: what changes do I need to make to my heat styling regimen?:

_____

_____

_____

Chemicals – what changes need to be made to my chemical processing? (decrease frequency, milder/stronger formula, etc)

_____

_____

_____

PART 4: Hair & scalp conditions (Chapter 5)

___ No, I am not experiencing dry, flaky scalp, split ends or splits in the hair shaft, knots at the ends, hair damage

___ Yes, I have one or more of the conditions listed above

___ Yes, I am experiencing hair loss (visit www.trichology.edu.au to find a local trichologist)

YOUR CUSTOMIZED HAIR HEALTH PLAN

ACTION PLAN:
If yes, what are the key changes I can make to improve the condition of my hair and scalp?

_____

_____

_____

PART 5:
Selecting Products (Chapter 6)
Which products need to be replaced or added to my hair care routine?

____ Hair Cleanser/Shampoo
____ Hair Conditioner
____ Leave-in moisturizer/conditioner
____ Shine Spray / Drops
____ Styling aid, what type: _____
____ Heat Protectant

As this book closes, I hope you will remember that it takes knowledge of the hair characteristics you have, willingness to know when you need to get help or make a change, and commitment to follow through on the steps you identify in your plan. Unfortunately, there are no magic pills or creams to transform your hair overnight. You will need to be patient and determined. If you experience a setback, don't give up. Finally, while your hair is part of your beauty, it will never be all you have to offer. Work towards beautiful, healthy hair as well as the best, healthiest you.

BONUS #1
CARING FOR CHILDREN'S HAIR

Although children can't be grouped into a single type for the purposes of learning about their hair, I wanted to include some guidance for care the development of good hair care practices. Like anything else you expose them to, good or bad, children learn to love or hate their hair from the way you handle theirs and yours. I transitioned from very long texturized hair to very short, very curly hair when my children were toddlers. After total frustration when dealing with a foreign hair texture (my own God given texture), I started to wear wigs and weaves exclusively. I used my hair as the anchor for either styling option. After several of years of this, I overheard my daughters asking each other "what kind of wig will you get when you get older?"

Each of my daughters has a full head of long, natural hair, but I was teaching them that my texture (and theirs) needed to be covered. This is just an example of how powerful our actions can be, even when we're not aware of the message we're sending or who may be listening.

I shared this experience to help you be more aware of how we shape the viewpoint a child may have about her own beauty. I also receive tons of questions about managing and using chemical processes on children's hair. For many with children of blended heritages, the child's hair is a texture different than both the father's and the mother's and quite possibly like no texture either parent has ever had to manage. If any of these situations describe you or someone you know, this part of the book will offer the information needed. So, let's start from the beginning.

Either an infant is born without hair and after birth grows their first cycle of very fine, unpigmented hair (lanugo), or others are born with up to an inch or two of straight or even curly hair.

Generally, this type of hair is very small in diameter and is easily managed with a mild "baby" shampoo. The hair can simply be rinsed with water during a bath and cleansed every few days unless it gets soiled. Typically, you are looking for a tear-free shampoo to avoid irritating the eyes. You will only need a dime to a nickel sized drop of shampoo. When washing the hair of an infant, be extremely gentle, remember to avoid pressure on the "soft spot" where the skull has not completely formed over the brain. After rinsing the hair thoroughly, gently pat the hair to remove excess moisture. Some infants experience dry hair, in these cases an application of a very small amount of pure olive oil will usually help resolve the dryness.

CRADLE CAP

This condition is the onset of seborrheic dermatitis in an infant. It will often appear as a yellow, crust-like formation on the scalp. The cause is generally believed to be an overgrowth of the natural yeast found on the scalp. It is not a sign of poor hygiene and generally harmless. If there is a small area affected, you can try daily shampoo and gentle massage of the area with pure olive oil (unless the "soft spot" is affected – no massage to this area). Rinse the excessive oil from the hair and shampoo again to remove any flakes that may have loosened. Let the flakes come loose in their own time, don't scratch them to speed up the process. Also, change the linens used on a daily basis until this resolves. If the cradle cap occurs in large areas on the scalp of extends to other parts of the body, see your pediatrician for treatment options.

Since babies are born with a relatively small amount of hair, some parents are anxious to showcase that their baby is a girl. There are tons of pretty headbands, barrettes, bows and clips that entice parents. Be careful that the headbands are not too tight and that they aren't worn for long periods of time. Headbands can break the fragile hair underneath. As for bows, barrettes, clips, etc., make sure they aren't pulling the hair to the point of stress. This means there should be some slack in the hair being pulled into the hair clamp. Again, you are trying to avoid breaking this fragile hair due to tension. If you are braiding the hair, make sure the braid can be slightly lifted from the hair to avoid traction damage. Be sure to take any of the clips out before the child goes to sleep to avoid injury or damage to the hair.

OTHER SCALP CONDITIONS

Aside from cradle cap, children may experience either tinea capitis (ringworm) or pediculosis capitis (lice). Both conditions are highly contagious.

Ringworm is caused by fungi that feed on keratin. Therefore, ringworm can feed on skin (soft keratin) or hard keratin (hair). An infection causes itchiness of the skin, inflammation and raised areas. If the hair is affected, the strand will often split or break easily. Dandruff shampoos containing selenium sulfide at 2.5-3% will help, but the child will need to see a doctor for prescription to resolve the infection.

Lice are another childhood nuisance. Here the eggs of the lice are being deposited in the hair at a rapid reproduction rate. The itching is severe and may cause additional infection. If you child is infected with lice, use commercial shampoos to address this. Follow the instructions diligently and see the pediatrician if the condition persists.

Remember, these conditions are highly contagious, so change linens, hats, clothing, etc. often and wash these items in hot water. Ensure the child isn't sharing hairbrushes or anything else that may come into contact with the infection. As a parent or caregiver, make sure you don't come into contact with the affected area.

AROUND 18 MONTHS / THE TODDLER YEARS:
You may notice the first texture change before or by the time your baby grows into an active toddler. Hair will likely increase in diameter and density, and start to accumulate more length. At this point, some frustration may set in as hair may start to tangle more than before.

The tangles are in part due to increased length and thickness, but mostly due to the rolling, sliding and active play that comes with this age. It can be tempting to heat straighten. Never give in to this quick fix. For those of us who grew up with hot combs and pressing oil, be aware that applying high heat and oil can cause the oil to contact and permanently scar the sensitive scalp of a child. Heat is a recipe for disaster and may cause permanent damage to your child's still developing hair pattern. As mentioned before, make sure your child doesn't sleep in barrettes, bows, etc.

Give your child the best chance of reaching adulthood with healthy hair. Working to change the hair texture (through heat or chemicals) and letting your child hear negative comments about his or her hair texture is damaging to the self-esteem of the child. These messages can be the foundation of not appreciating the features that he or she has. As a parent or caregiver, you are the main line of defense to protect your child from these kinds of experiences.

CHEMICALS:
DON'T, under any circumstances, chemically process the hair of a child under age 12. The reason is that they will undergo another texture change around puberty. I get asked all the time about "kiddie perms". These are the same relaxers adults get but with lower percentages of the active ingredients. The odds of overprocessing or getting a chemical burn are extremely high. Ever tried to get a kid to stop scratching a mosquito bite? It will be as hard (or harder) to prevent scratching before a relaxer or chemical treatment. I know there are many people who have relaxed children's hair with beautiful results, but I know many who wish they had never done so. Don't put your child in the position to one day be the adult who says, "I had thick, long hair as a child..."

So what should you do? You're dealing with manageability issues, so let's talk about strategies to make this process as painless as possible.

TANGLES – childhood hair enemy #1
Tangles are bundles of hairs that get wrapped around each other. There are two primary ways to attack this problem, either mechanically and chemically (with products, not chemical treatments/processing).
Mechanically, keep hairs from rubbing against each other.

At night, comb through hair to remove tangles. Start at the ends with a wide tooth comb and a good detangling product. Most detangling products contain humectants to moisturize hair which makes it less likely to "flyaway," and a lower pH to close the cuticle and minimize hairs catching on one another. Some people prefer to detangle by hand and skip a comb, if you want to hand detangle go to step 2.

1) Select your detangling comb. What is a wide tooth comb? The concept here is to use the comb with the widest distance between teeth to do the first pass of detangling. Once that is complete, you can move to the next smaller width for better alignment of hair.

The teeth of the combs are spaced as follows:

| | - Wide tooth comb
| | - Medium width comb spacing
| | - Small tooth comb
|| - Rat tail comb spacing (only for straight hair that has been detangled)

2) Once you've selected the comb needed, start about an inch above the ends. Comb downwards but immediately stop if the comb catches a mass of hairs. If this happens, gently separate the mass by hand.

3) Resume detangling by going up another inch above where you started and repeat the downward combing process.

4) Continue until the you have reached the roots and can glide the wide tooth comb effortlessly through the hair to the ends.

Is this process time consuming? Absolutely, but without it you will find that the tangles build until you have massive areas of tangling.

What if you don't have time for this on a daily basis? Recognize that letting your child wear their hair loose will encourage tangles, you may want to consider alternate styles that do more to protect hair from tangles. Consider having your child's hair sectioned and braided into pigtails or 2-strand twists. These options are very child appropriate and prevent playtime from becoming tangle-time. In addition to a good detangling process and protective styling, the right products can be a huge help.

SHAMPOOS/CONDITIONER

Once your child transitions into his or her first texture change, then it's time to determine their hair type as we covered in Chapter 3. The baby shampoo is no longer appropriate for most hair types and may cause severe dryness for those with curly/wavy hair types. Also, conditioner is a must for the new texture. See product selection tips from chapter 6 for more details.

For those parents who have children of blended heritages, if the hair is more dense, curlier or wavier than yours, your shampoo will likely not be appropriate for his or her hair type. The child will also likely need leave-in moisturizers and perhaps even pomade to keep from having dry, frizzy curls. Also, daily hair washing is too frequent and will dry hair out. Try once or twice a week should be sufficient unless the hair gets soiled.

Shampoo & Conditioner Process:

It is vital to perform the cleansing and conditioning steps to avoid the tangles in the first place. If you can safely place the child on the kitchen counter and use the kitchen sink with the sprayer attachment, it may make this process much easier.

1) Have the child lay on his or her back on the counter. (using a waterproof sleep mat or placing a blanket inside a large trash bag, may make the

counter more comfortable)

2) Direct all hair back into the sink and away from the face.

3) Adjust the water so it is warm and comfortable to the child. Periodically check to make sure the water temp isn't creeping up or down.

4) Thoroughly wet all the hair, keeping it straight and in the sink away from the child's face and neck.

5) Once all hair is wet, gently squeeze out some of the excess water. Extra water will dilute your shampoo/cleanser causing you to use more than is needed.

6) Apply shampoo/cleanser to your hands, then rub them together. Reach into the child's hair and apply the shampoo to the scalp throughout the hair. Gently massage the scalp all over. You may need more shampoo for the back of the scalp. You will start to see that the shampoo/cleanser is making its way down the length of the hair, if not, apply more product to your hands and smooth it down the hair shaft towards the ends. Be sure to not pile the hair on the scalp and slide it around – this can cause damage to the hair and introduce tangles.

7) Rinse the hair thoroughly after cleansing

8) Squeeze out excess moisture, apply conditioner throughout the hair, even if you have to lift sections and reapply. Conditioner can't treat what it does not touch. Note that conditioner is generally for the hair, so there is no need to massage it into the scalp.

9) Follow the instructions on your conditioner. Rinse conditioner out thoroughly, again keeping hair as straight as possible.

10) Gently squeeze excess moisture from the hair and wrap a towel around the hair before you take the child down from the counter. Be careful not to

rub the towel back and forth to dry hair. Instead, use the towel to gently squeeze out excessive moisture. With each step, focus on keeping the hairs from rubbing together.

11) Apply your detangling product and/or leave-in moisturizer.

12) Divide the hair into four sections and proceed to detangle.

Yes, there are a lot of steps, but giving your child the best chance for beautiful, healthy hair is worth the effort.

Chlorine & Salt

Most kids love to take advantage of every chance they get to swim in a pool. If there is chlorine or saltwater, take care to protect the hair using these simple steps.

1) Thoroughly wet hair before getting in the pool or saltwater

2) Apply a light-weight leave-in conditioner

The theory here is that pre-dampened and conditioned hair will not absorb as much chlorinated/salt water since it is already wet. The leave-in protects hair. Of course, you should still shampoo and condition hair after swimming.

For blondes, the steps are the same and may help prevent the "green" tone that comes from the reaction of copper in the water with the hair.

Before we close, let's take a closer look at the styling options you have and the best ways to avoid damage.

Pigtails/ponytails: These are great options for kids when done correctly. There are 2 key considerations:

1) Tension – whether you do one or many ponytails, make sure none of them are too tight. Remember, at this age, the hairline and entire perimeter of hair (over the ears and around to the nape) is still growing in. Too much tension on these fragile

areas can cause traction alopecia and result in permanent hair loss over time. Edge control, as we discussed, is often a major focus in children's hair care (avoiding "kitchens" – curly hair at the nape that some consider to be unsightly and slicking down "baby hair" in the front). These types of practices break fragile hair.

2) Placement – be creative with how you section and place the ponytails. Hair held in the same way can develop permanent parts – which really means you have trained the hair to separate and be directed a certain way.

Braids/twists: Again, high tension must be avoided. Be especially mindful of this with professional braiders. Many are focusing on capturing every strand of hair and making perfect braids/twists. Anytime your scalp hurts, it's an indicator that your follicle is being traumatized. Trauma to the follicle is a great way to damage it and lose the hair.

Extensions- many people love the look of long flowing hair, even on children. There are some points to keep in mind here:

1) Along with the tension of the twist or braid, the extra hair is extra weight on the hair follicle. When you double or triple the length of your hair, the follicle is getting a lot of stress.

2) With the natural hair entwined with extension hair, it can be hard to keep your child's hair clean, conditioned and properly moisturized. Using synthetic hair can be even more damaging than human hair. At the very least, don't leave extensions in for months at a time.

Trimming/cutting hair:

There are old wives tail that cutting a child's hair before they turn a year old will cause texture problems or letting your cut hair get taken by a bird who builds a nest with it will cause texture issues as well.

Needless to say, these are ridiculous. Hair is comprised of dead cells which means the ends of the hair cannot transmit messages back to the follicle. In fact, your child's hair undergoes abuse that goes way beyond what some adults experience from playing, to napping, rolling on the floor, etc. and as a result, split ends can occur in their hair as well. Although growth of a child's hair may be important to the parent, as we discussed earlier, split ends don't correct themselves. If you aren't comfortable with trimming damaged ends, find a stylist who can do so and maintain as much length as possible. Be clear if you are not seeking to make hair even throughout (that plan yields a lot more trimming).

In conclusion, take time to nurture your child's hair and his or her thoughts about the hair. The gift of beautiful, healthy hair may be one of the most valuable steps in establishing good self-esteem.

Angela Adams McGhee

BONUS #2
Selecting Tools for Great Haircare

In order to help with styling, there are a few styling tools that will be very helpful.

1) Combs – it is very important to choose a comb of good quality. If the comb is plastic, test that it is rigid and that there are no burrs of seams in the comb. These imperfections are more than enough to damage the cuticle of the hair strand. You may want to choose several combs since they serve different purposes.

The teeth of the combs are spaced as follows:

| | | - Wide tooth comb – best for detangling of high density, curly/wavy hair types

| | | - Medium width comb spacing – best for detangling of med/low density; small diameter hair

| | - Small tooth comb – best for alignment of small diameter, low density hair

|| - Rat tail comb spacing – the "tail" of this comb is very effective in creating precision parts in all types, the teeth should only be used in small diameter, straight hair.

2) BRUSHES:

Boar bristles are the widely recognized standard in hair brushes. They are available in a wide variety of styles from baby soft to stiff. Use only the very softest brush bristles on infants. As texture changes, use only the level of stiffness needed to move your hair. By now, everyone should know that brushing your hair 100 times each day is just a way to erode the cuticle and damage the hair. Brushing can help distribute sebum down the hair shaft, but this is generally only effective for those with straight hair or with large waves. Most in the curly/wavy texture types omit a brush all together because brushing separates ringlets which causes frizz.

The really stiff bristled brushes are best used by African-American men who are "training" very short hair to follow a wave pattern.

3) ELASTIC BANDS

Rubber bands are best used as an office supply. For the hair, look for stretchy fabric bands that don't have metal clasps. The metal can be damaging to hair once it is wound tightly .

4) CUTTING SHEARS:

These are very sharp scissors designated only for cutting hair (not the pesky plastic tag on your clothes or anything else). To get a good pair, visit your local beauty supply store. Test them by opening and closing the blades a few times. There should be no drag or hesitation in closing the blades. Ice-tempered is one designation that provides a very good cut. Remember to keep these out of the reach of children at all times. They will easily cut open a finger (especially a small one), but are needed to give the hair strand a good, clean cut. Using dull scissors on hair encourages split ends.

5) SATIN SLEEP CAPS/WRAPS
OR PILLOWCASES

I am a true believer in the benefit of protecting hair during sleep. The tossing and turning will wreck your style, tangle and damage your hair. Look for caps that have a flat band that isn't too tight. Your entire hairline should be inside the cap. If you prefer a satin scarf, again, ensure the hairline is enclosed. Wrap all hair so that it stays inside the scarf. Needless to say, don't over tighten the scarf. For those who can't endure anything on your head, a satin pillowcase will help. I would also recommend protective styling (like loose braids or banding to make sure you don't introduce masses of tangles).

6) BLOW DRYERS/CURLING/FLAT IRONS

For blow dryers, wattage determines the amount of heat it can produce. Most models are rated at 1875 Watts. The differentiating factor after that would be the types of internal components. Most professionals use dryers with ceramic and/or tourmaline inside plates. Ceramic is valued for its ability to disperse and hold heat consistently. Tourmaline is believed to produce ions that help hair dry faster. Likewise, in flat irons, these materials are used. Ceramic for even heating across the plates that contact the hair. Tourmaline for production of ions believed to smooth the hair cuticle. While these may help you select a good blow dryer or flat iron, be sure to keep the heat at 350 degrees, cover small sections, and use heat protectant as previously discussed to best reduce possible damage to hair.

Angela Adams McGhee

BONUS #3
Transitioning to Natural Hair

For those who are planning to discontinue relaxer services, texturizers, or any other texture altering services, this section is for you. If it has been awhile since you last interacted with your natural texture, you will need to revisit chapter 4 to determine the characteristics of the new growth and develop a plan to ensure healthy growth in chapter 7. Many transitioners consider growing hair out to a certain length then cutting off the chemically processed ends. This method can be effective provided you understand that you will need to be extremely gentle with the hair due to the weakness of the hair at the union of the two different textures. Keep in mind that the new growth must be well conditioned, moisturized, and detangled on a regular basis to avoid loc formation in the new growth. Keeping the processed hair and new growth in similar textures may help prevent breakage. For example, two-strand twists or twist-outs give wavy texture to the entire length of the strand. Thermally straightening hair will also make the new growth and processed hair more closely match in terms of texture.

If this process seems too daunting, other transitioners opt for the "big chop" where all the processed hair is cut off at once. Before deciding to do this type of transition, consider how you will style and care for your hair. Many find that two-strand twists or twist-outs are a great way to style relatively short new growth. Using good detangling practices (pg. 76) and the Moisture Sealing Process (pg. 18) will give your hair the moisture and hold it needs to create twists that don't readily unravel. Wearing wigs during transition is also a possibility, but don't neglect the hair underneath.

The one piece of advice I give anyone who transitions is to be prepared for the solicited and unsolicited comments. Whether it is a co-worker, family member or significant other, many people find the concept of natural, unprocessed hair uncomfortable. In response, you may hear very negative comments or be showered with compliments. The main idea is to be aware that not everyone may embrace the emergence of your new texture. If that is your experience, remind yourself of the reasons you chose to transition. Be prepared to be patient. As you adjust to your natural texture, remember that hormonal changes, and length of hair can affect your curl pattern. Be observant to changes and adjust your Customized Hair Health Plan each time you experience changes in your hair.

REFERENCES

(1)-(3)
The Hair and Scalp ©1993, David Salinger, IAT
   International Association of Trichologists

(4)
Dietary Reference Intakes for Energy, Carbohydrate, Fiber,
   Fat, Fatty Acids, Cholesterol, Protein, and Amino
   Acids. Washington, D.C.: National Academies
   Press, ©2005.

(5)
Nutrition ©1999, David Salinger, IAT
   International association of Trichologists

Angela Adams McGhee

ABOUT THE AUTHOR

Angela Adams McGhee was born in Memphis, Tennessee. She attended Florida A&M University where she majored in chemistry and received a bachelor's of science in the subject. She founded Definitive Formulations in 2004. Definitive Formulations is a manufacturer of customized hair care, skin care, and fragrance products for the private label market used by salons and boutiques across the country. In 2014, she became a certified trichologist through the Internal Association of Trichologists. In 2015, she began Definitive Trichology. She helps clients re-grow and maintain healthy hair. In addition, she periodically teaches classes through the University of Central Arkansas.

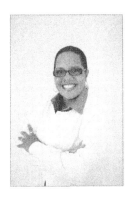

Angela Adams McGhee

INDEX

Printed in Great Britain
by Amazon